Carnivore Diet 101 for Beginners

The Ultimate Carnivore Diet Guide

John Caldwell

Introduction

Are you tired of having tasteless veggie meals through and through to lose weight but it seems not to be working?

Do want to enjoy your favorite meat-based meals while remaining healthy and fit?

Are you looking for a simple-to-follow meal plan that doesn't require you to have a chef's skills?

If yes, this is the book for you.

There are multiple diets out there that promise to help you lose weight and improve your wellbeing. However, many require you to spend a lot of time in the kitchen preparing and cooking or are challenging to keep up with, or they only include salads and vegetable smoothies that, honestly, taste and smell weird.

Well, not the carnivore diet. With this eating approach, you are allowed all the varieties of meat out there, which you can prepare however you like. Are you ready to embark on this simple high protein all meat-eating style and enjoy all the benefits that come along with it?

In this book, we will cover:

- What is the carnivore diet
- Varieties of the carnivore diet
- Foods to eat and avoid on the diet
- Getting started
- The benefits and side effects
- Frequently asked questions
- A carnivore diet meal plan and recipes

And so much more!

Let's dive right in!

Table of Contents

Chapter 1: What is The Carnivore Diet?

Also known as the "all-meat diet," this diet focuses on the consumption of just animal-based foods such as fish, meat, and a selection of dairy. It aims at restricting the intake of carbs to the lowest possible point (typically zero carbs) while focussing on eating more fat and protein.

How the Carnivore Diet Works

Most low-carb diets tend to restrict most plant-based options since carbohydrates come from plants. The most stringent low-carb meal plan the carnivore diet, emphasizes elimination of all plant-based foods, including seeds, nuts, and non-starchy veggies common on other similar diet plans such as paleo, keto, and Atkins. Carbohydrates are not a crucial nutrient despite the widespread belief, which means that we do not require them to function appropriately and survive. Nevertheless, this does not imply that we are essentially meant to survive with no carbs.

Like the keto diet, this meal plan promotes a state of ketosis as you switch from sugars as the primary energy source for your body to fat (ketones). However, with this diet, the ketosis state is not required, and it is not as central as it is with the keto diet. Due to this, it is advisable to consume sufficient high-fat animal-based foods to keep your energy levels up.

Let us now move on to what to eat and drink while on the carnivore diet:

What to Eat and Drink on The Carnivore Diet

As its name suggests, this meal plan is extreme where you can eat fish and meat. There are several versions of the diet, and each of these distinctions has varying suggestions of the foods you should eat and avoid.

Versions of carnivore diet include:

- Keto carnivore
- Modified
- Standard
- Strict

As for the beverages, it is recommended that you drink bone broth and plenty of water but restrict the intake of coffee, tea, veggie juice, fruit juice, and, most importantly, alcohol.

Strict Carnivore Diet Food List

When you follow this version of the carnivore meal plan, you can have any meat, fish, and poultry, including organ meats such as intestines, brain, and liver, as well as bone marrow.

Below is the list of foods allowed on this variation:

- All fish and meat
- Bone broth
- Organ meats
- Eggs
- Poultry
- Shellfish
- Pork rinds
- Jerky (without added sugar)
- Tallow
- Lard

Foods You Should Avoid

- Processed foods
- Grains
- Nuts and seeds
- Vegetables
- Fruits
- Dairy: butter, cheese, yogurt, milk
- Vegetable oils
- Sweetened beverages
- Coffee and tea
- Alcohol
- Sugar

Standard Carnivore Diet Food List

This interpretation of the carnivore diet usually permits some low-carb, high-fat dairy products in addition to all meats.

The foods allowed include:

- Bone broth
- All meat and fish
- Bone marrow
- Organ meats
- Eggs
- Poultry
- Shellfish
- Jerky (no added sugar)
- Pork rinds
- Tallow
- Lard
- High-fat dairy such as kefir, hard cheeses, ghee cream, butter, yogurt

Foods To Avoid

- Processed foods
- Sugar
- Grains
- Vegetables
- Nuts and seeds
- Vegetable oils
- Sweetened Beverages
- Tea and coffee
- Fruits
- Alcohol

Modified Carnivore Diet Food List

On this variation of the carnivore diet, small quantities of particular plant foods low in sugar, such as cucumber, lettuce, and avocado, are allowed.

The Foods Allowed Include:

- Poultry
- All meat and fish
- Low carb dairy: cottage cheese, kefir, cheese, ghee cream, butter, yogurt
- Non-starchy veggies: onion, celery, radish, lettuce, cucumbers
- Shellfish
- Vegetable oils
- Avocado
- Tea and coffee
- Jerky (no added sugar)
- Tallow
- Bone broth
- Organ meats

- Lard
- Pork rinds
- Bone marrow
- Eggs

Foods to Avoid Include:

- Sweetened Beverages
- Nuts and seeds
- Alcohol
- Processed foods
- Fruits
- Grains
- Most Vegetables
- Sugar

Keto Carnivore Diet Food List

The keto variation of the carnivore meal plan permits more plant foods approved in the keto diet and non-starchy veggies, seeds, and nuts. This carnivore diet is basically the keto diet with more emphasis on fish and meat.

Foods Allowed Include:

- Low carb dairy: cottage cheese, kefir, cheese, ghee cream, butter, yogurt
- Pork rinds
- All meat and fish
- Avocado
- Bone broth
- Tallow
- Vegetable oils
- Organ meats

- Non-starchy veggies: onion, celery, radish, lettuce, cucumbers
- Nuts and seeds
- Poultry
- Shellfish
- Jerky (no added sugar)
- Tea and coffee
- Bone marrow
- Lard
- Eggs

Foods to Avoid Include:

- Starchy Vegetables
- Sweetened Beverages
- Alcohol
- Grains
- Fruits
- Sugar

So how what do you stand to benefit by embracing the carnivore diet?

Chapter 2: Benefits of Embracing The Carnivore Diet

The following are the benefits of going carnivore:

Weight Loss

As much as low-carb meal plans are progressively gaining popularity as a weight-loss tool, it's not necessarily the restriction of carbs that make them successful. In the end, losing weight occurs due to the lowered intake of calories, and sometimes, diets that are low in carbs make it seem easier.

This happens due to a combination of reduced calorie intake and decreased hunger. Protein is the primary nutrient of the carnivore diet and is discerned as very satisfying. An increase in your protein intake is linked to improved calorie control, fewer cravings, and decreased hunger. Moreover, protein helps in improving body composition, which in turn aids in supporting lean muscle mass.

Typically, a high protein meal plan offers 30-40% calories from protein, while a carnivore one can double that. Additionally, when you restrict whole nutrient groups such as carbohydrates, it seriously moderates the types of food you can eat and helps you to stay on track with your goals. Also, carbs especially tend to be conveniently present in options that are not nutritious in the form of added sugars and refined grains. Therefore, when we completely cut off carbs from our diet, it often means removing most of the additional calories from beverages, sweets, and snacks, leading to reduced body weight and lesser intake of calories.

Improved Mental Clarity

Similar to the Keto diet, the carnivore approach presents several metabolic modifications to bodily processes. The body starts using ketones for fuel from readily available glucose. Whereas most assume that easily accessible fuel is more suitable for the brain, the truth is actually the opposite. The thing about glucose is that your body undergoes constant fluctuations of troughs and peaks. Although, once it adjusts to ketones, the body breaks down fat from your meals or the stored fat in your body. While on a carnivore or keto diet, it is those ketones that provide enhanced mental focus

Simple Meal Plan

If you have attempted various meal plans and other eating approaches to aid in weight loss, you know that dieting can sometimes get complicated.

A carnivore meal plan is entirely different. If the product is sourced from an animal, then it's basically on the table. As you advance into the diet, it will call for a bit more restriction; do not overthink it though.

Before you get started with the carnivore diet, let us at look some risks and how to deal with them so that you are prepared.

Let us now move on to how to get started on the carnivore diet:

Chapter 3: Getting Started on the Carnivore Diet

The thing about this diet is that you eat until you feel full; sounds easy enough. Meat is a phenomenal filler, and it's sure going to surprise you with the little it takes to sustain you for several hours. This way, you do not have to keep snacking, and you can actually lose weight.

On average, you should eat approximately 2 pounds of meat per day. However, during the first month, you may be consuming a lot more while you battle craving other foods and as your appetite and digestive system adjust. Once your body adjusts, you can begin tracking your activity and calories for weight loss.

Then it comes down to whether you simply want to lose a couple of pounds or build muscle; if you work out daily at the gym and would like to bulk up, consuming 4 pounds or more is suitable.

When To Eat

Eat as much as you require and as often as you need to feel satisfied. If you prefer spreading your meals out throughout the day, three meals should do the trick. Alternatively, you can add some periods of fasting and go with a meal or 2 in a day. Having said that, it is generally advisable to stick to 3 meals a day.

Approximately two weeks into this meal plan, your metabolism will adapt to being additionally efficient at acquiring energy from fats. This suggests that you should also include the fatty cuts of meat since you have to consume animal meat/fat to power your brain and body; in the same way as on the keto diet.

Begin your day with a nice fix of protein, then maintain the protein levels throughout your day. This is particularly vital if you are attempting to manage your body weight, build muscle or work out at the gym daily.

Where to Get Your Meat

Local Butcher

No one will support and understand your carnivore meal plan better than your neighborhood butcher. Butchers are equipped with vast knowledge of various animal cuts. Since you will be purchasing meat in large quantities, also expect them to welcome you with enthusiasm.

Farmers' Market

Before starting the carnivore diet, it's a pretty good idea to note when the farmers' market in your area takes place. It's among the top spots to get exceptionally fresh red meat. Suppliers at these places mainly provide pasture-raised and grass-fed animal products, which means more nutritional value for you.

Supermarkets

If your budget for the carnivore diet feels stretched, try checking out the section of pre-packed meat or the butcher area at the supermarket. It's not the most suitable option, and it can be challenging to get the rarer cuts or sections; however, it's always a choice.

Buying Online

It is now possible to purchase your meat online. We have numerous meat delivery services providing safe methods, including Snake River Farms, Amazon, ButcherBox, Kansas City Steak, Porter Road, US Wellness Meat, and many more. Most of these services offer grass-fed frozen and fresh meat.

Things to Consider Before Getting Started on The Carnivore Diet

Before you can jump into this eating lifestyle, there are a couple of things you'll have to consider. Let's dive in!

Not Eating Plants

Avoiding plant-based foods is way more intricate than it may appear, even for the greatest fans of BBQ and meat. If you have tried keeping a food journal before, you will notice how frequently you add snacks such as a banana, an apple, or a granola bar.

You also won't be having your afternoon coffee nor a cookie. A carnivore diet is all about steering clear of any carbs and primarily consuming meat.

Drinking More Water and Hot Beverages

The importance of water on a carnivore diet cannot be stressed enough. You need to drink 5 pints of water daily. In standard plant and meat-based diets with lots of vegetables and fruits, the foods contain plenty of water, meaning that when you switch to a carnivore diet, which is only meat-based, it dramatically reduces most of your liquid intake. Even if your meat is rare to medium, most of the liquid contained evaporates during cooking. Try having a whole pint of carnivore-allowed beverages with each of your meals; after that, just spread out two more pints. It's that simple.

You can also drink tea and coffee, including herbal teas, so long as they are not sweetened with any sugar. You will need to stay away from any drink containing carbs such as energy drinks, vegetable and fruit juices, and soda since they will keep you from achieving your weight loss goals.

If you do not like the taste of plain water and cannot imagine yourself drinking water throughout your day, it would be a good idea to include hot beverages. Remember that you will need to up your fluid intake when you take coffee since caffeine dehydrates the body. Alternatively, you could skip the coffee and invest in the various ranges of herbal teas that are free of caffeine. For example, green tea is advantageous for you as it contains a good amount of antioxidants- though it may be an acquired taste.

How to Cook the Meat

As a beginner on an all-meat diet, it is advisable to keep to your usual taste. If rare is how you prefer your beef, you are already enjoying the most advantages since the less you cook your meat, the less protein that gets destroyed by the heat. Though if you have been eating your beef well-done, continue with that for the time being and slowly adjust to rarer meat.

For poultry and pork, ensure that you cook them thoroughly (for your safety and health) while at the same time avoiding getting it dried out entirely. To be on the safe side, try using a meat thermometer such as *ThermoPro TP20* so that you cook your meat right every time.

It is safe to eat most fish raw though it might be an acquired taste. Just attempt it and if it doesn't agree with you, cook it the way you prefer.

You can eat all kinds of meat

Do not just ask your butcher for striploin steaks and pork chops. Switch things up frequently between fresh fish, lamb, pork, organ meat, and beef. When you switch between different meats every day, it ensures that you boost your uptake of minerals and vitamins. This also ensures that your body gets everything it requires by getting the complete variety of amino acids.

Athletes Need to Be Patient to Get Results

During the first several weeks, high-performance athletes might have a hard time. This is because the body is not getting quick energy from glucose, which comes from carbs. The body will instead require to adjust to breaking down more fat. It is important to note that it is not about the lack of calories but rather the kind of calorie ingestion you are now partaking. Improvements in both mental and physical drive will begin to manifest. For other athletes, there can be an exception. They may need to add a few plant-based foods during the first weeks to maintain the levels of raw energy and operate at their best.

Now that you are ready to adopt this diet, it is important to know the different levels of embracing the carnivore diet:

Chapter 4: The Different Levels of the Carnivore Diet

It can be very overwhelming to make sudden extreme changes to your diet. Therefore we will look at three levels you can work through as you get started.

The Levels of Adapting

The different levels you can work through as you begin are:

Level 1

The rule of thumb for this level is that any meat belongs to a plate. There are no strict guidelines yet on the level of processing or the type of cuts or meat. You can also have coffee and tea, cheese, butter, full-fat cream, and eggs, just to provide a bit of diversity as you ease into the diet.

You are also allowed some electrolyte supplements, pepper, and table salt that help in reducing any effects of dehydration and making the food taste more recognizable to your taste buds.

Don't get me wrong; this level is still a drastic adjustment, though not as much as the last level. It simply allows you the chance to adapt mentally and physically.

Level 2

After being in the first level for about 2-4 weeks, you are now ready for the second level, where all non-meat products are not allowed. From a dietetic point of view, you will only be ingesting water and meat. Any meats that are highly processed, such as salami and pastrami, should also be avoided. Dairy products too. You can still use pepper and salt but in moderation. The concept of this level is taking a further step in becoming an actual carnivore dieter.

Level 3

After you have spent 2-4 more weeks on the second level, the next step would be the third level, where you'll only be allowed to have grass-fed beef and no other meat. Feel free to alternate between different cuts of beef as desired and organ meats too from a cow. Sure this will be significantly costlier. However, the nutrient richness and quality of pasture beef are way more superior. If this becomes overly high priced for you, you can avoid poultry, fish, and pork and stick to beef.

Beyond Level 3

You will remain in the third level for around 30 days, after which you begin observing changes in your metabolism and digestion; you'll start to notice things such as increased mental and physical energy.

During this step, you can occasionally throw in some of the foods that were restricted in the second and third levels. To help in staying motivated, you can try taking common alternatives such as seafood and lamb. Nevertheless, make sure to stick to eating grass-fed beef mostly. The point is to get you to recognize the sources of meat that make you feel sick or bloated to make your carnivore experience as comfortable as possible for you. In the end, you should have gathered a whole list of all-meat products that you can stick with.

Selecting The Level to Begin With

Generally, it is recommended to begin with the first level. However, if you are not addicted to caffeine, you can start with level 2. It is not advised to begin with the third level as you will indeed have a hard time with the new carnivore limitations. Also, try spending a minimum of 30 days between the first and second levels before taking the last step.

Surviving The First Month of the Carnivore Diet

Before getting started on this meal plan, it is crucial to understand how difficult the first month (particularly week 1) will be. You will be changing your entire style of eating. Therefore, your body will take some time to adjust. Below are a few things to take note of for your transitioning to be easier:

Have Your Blood Tested

Before beginning the carnivore diet, make sure to get your blood work, and then again roughly 2 months into the diet. Each person has distinct metabolic requirements; thus, it's critical to discern whether the diet is in harmony with your body.

It can be far better and easier working with a physician.

Don't give up when you feel sickly

In the first week of the carnivore diet, you are more likely to experience headaches, fatigue, and other flu-like symptoms. Don't worry, as it's a typical stage of the procedure as the body acclimatizes to getting energy from fats instead of carbs.

Expect Fluctuations in Your Appetite

There are some days where you will not even be thinking about food and other days where you will feel like eating non-stop. Once the body familiarizes with the diet, your appetite will stabilize as well.

Chapter 5: Common Mistakes to Avoid On the Carnivore Diet

When starting, don't be overly confident about how easy it may sound to stick to eating just meat. I mean, how can you mess up prepping the meat and eating? Well, there happens to be several things you should avoid on this meal plan, and they include:

Sneaking some veggies and fruit

When some get into the diet, they think that so long as red meat is their primary food source, it's okay to do this, but that's not the case; it lowers your chances of getting into ketosis. There's a reason why this diet is referred to as a meat-based diet – just stick to eating meat.

Purchasing lean cuts only

All meat comes in fatty and lean cuts. This doesn't mean that you should eat pork belly daily; however, don't fear eating fat as it's what fuels your body.

Drinking too little water

Many veggies and fruits are usually high in water so even if you do not take as much water in the normal diet, you can still get some water from fruits and veggies. With this diet, you do not eat fruits and veggies; hence, you cannot get any water from this foods. Thus, it is important to increase your intake of water.

Not Eating Enough

The carnivore diet requires that you eat to your feel. The good news is that meat is quite filling so you would not have to eat a lot to feel satisfied.

Not Adding Salt

Electrolytes are crucial for your blood's salinity. When your diet only comprises meat, there is a sudden significant reduction in salts, so make sure to include it in your meals as a seasoning, but in moderation.

Chapter 6: Risks Associated with The Carnivore Diet

Below are the potential risks of this diet:

High in Fat, Sodium, and Cholesterol

If the version you choose consists entirely of animal foods, it may be higher in cholesterol and saturated fat. Consuming high amounts of saturated fat can raise LDL levels (bad cholesterol), which can promote chances of developing heart disease.

Also, some meats that are processed, particularly breakfast meats and bacon, are high in sodium. Consuming much of these meats on a carnivore meal plan may result in an excessive intake of sodium, which has previously been associated with a higher chance of promoting kidney disease, high blood pressure, and other health-related risks.

Therefore, it would be best to adopt the strict carnivore diet for a shorter period.

May Lack Particular Beneficial Plant Compounds And Micronutrients

As we mentioned before, this diet restricts highly nutritious food stuffs such as whole grains, legumes, vegetables, and fruits, all of which comprise advantageous minerals and vitamins. As much as meat offers micronutrients and is very nutritious, it shouldn't be the sole item on your menu. Sticking to restrictive diets such as a carnivore meal plan can result in overconsumption of some nutrients and deficiencies in others. When you remove carbs from your diet altogether, you remove chief sources of major nutrients such as fiber, potassium, Vitamin E, Vitamin A, and Vitamin C.

Moreover, meal plans abundant in plant-based foods have been linked to reduced chances of developing specific chronic issues such as type

2 diabetes, Alzheimer's, certain cancers, and heart disease. This is not entirely due to the high content of minerals, fiber, and vitamins in plant meals but also their antioxidants and valuable plant compounds.

Sure, fish and meat offer rich nutrition and are an exceptional supply of quality protein. However, they can't provide all the necessary minerals and vitamins required by your body to thrive and function well.

Thus, the need to include some plant compounds occasionally to ensure that you do not experience any deficiencies.

Does Not Offer Fiber

Fiber is the non-digestible carbohydrate that supports healthy bowel movements and gut health; it's only found in plant-based foods. Therefore, since the carnivore is an all-meat diet, it doesn't include any fiber, leading to constipation in some people.

Also, fiber is crucial in appropriately balancing bacteria in your gut. When your gut health is suboptimal, it causes several issues, and it can be associated with weakening of immunity and colon cancer.

According to a study done on low carb, high protein diet, 17 men with obesity were found to have considerably lower levels of the components which aid in protecting against colon cancer, in contrast to moderate carb, high protein diets.

Generally, sticking to a carnivore diet in the long-term may not be the best idea.

It Might Not be Ideal for Some People

For some people, following a carnivore meal plan can be particularly problematic. For instance, people who require limiting their protein intake, such as those with chronic kidney disease, must not attempt following this diet.

Additionally, hyper-responders to cholesterol or those that are extra susceptible to cholesterol in their meals should take caution in eating foods rich in cholesterol.

Also, if you are pregnant or breastfeeding as well as children and people who have special nutritional intake requirements, this diet may not be suitable for you. Finally, the carnivore diet is not recommended for people who have a hard time with restrictive eating or have anxiety about food.

Chapter 7: Carnivore Diet FAQ`

Is it dangerous to only eat protein?

No, it is not. Your body is also ingesting macros such as fat and many vitamins and minerals. An absolute carnivore diet accompanied by an active lifestyle will offer many advantages brought about by a ketogenic metabolism, which we discussed above.

Which is the healthiest meat?

Generally, grass-fed and organic meat is the most nourishing. It is always best to opt for certified organic when you are interested in following an all-meat diet. It is better to go for less expensive organic cuts instead of the costlier popular cuts.

Is it okay to only eat chicken?

No, it's not. This is because chicken does not comprise an adequate balance of micro-nutrition; therefore, you won't be getting most of the vitamins required by your body.

Can you only eat fish?

No, it's not advisable to only have fish as it also does not offer an adequate balance of protein and fat, which will result in undesirable outcomes. Fish provides many advantages, such as a wide range of vitamins and plenty of omega fatty acids. Nevertheless, the body will need other nutrients that are not present in fish.

Chapter 8: Carnivore Diet Meal Plan

As mentioned earlier, it is recommended to ease into the carnivore diet using the 3-level strategy until you work your way to eating just beef. The meal plan below will steadily alter the selection of meat over the first 4 weeks until you reach the third level.

Week 1 Diet Plan

For your first week on the carnivore meal plan, you will notice a couple of dairy items that you can still enjoy. This helps you to not feel deprived.

Monday

Breakfast: 5 slices (about 4 ounces) of bacon and 1-2 (3 ounces) 100% pork sausages

Lunch: The grilled beef burger patty only (10 ounces) with a slice of cheese

Dinner: Four fresh racks of lamb (12 ounces)

Tuesday

Breakfast: 3 (5 ounces) grilled pork sausages, 3 slices (4 ounces) of bacon

Lunch: Roasted salmon cutlets on the bone (15 ounces) with butter

Dinner: Grilled porterhouse steak (12 ounces) with butter

Wednesday

Breakfast: Grilled trout fillets (10 ounces) with butter

Lunch: Roasted pork belly (10 ounces)

Dinner: Slow roast topside of beef (12 ounces)

Thursday

Breakfast: Ground beef burger patty- grilled with some cheese

Lunch: Roast salmon (15 ounces) with butter

Dinner: Grilled porterhouse steak (12 ounces)

Friday

Breakfast: 2 grilled chicken breasts with skin (8 ounces)

Lunch: Grilled trout fillets (16 ounces)

Dinner: Slow roast topside of beef (12 ounces)

Saturday

Breakfast: 3 (5 ounces) grilled 100% pork sausages, 3 slices (4 ounces) of bacon

Lunch: 4 lamb chops (12 ounces)

Dinner: Grilled ribeye steak (12 ounces)

Sunday

Breakfast: 2 (8 ounces) grilled chicken breasts with skin

Lunch: 4 (12 ounces) pork chops fried or grilled

Dinner: Grilled ribeye steak (12 ounces)

Week 1 Shopping List

Topside of beef: 24 ounces

Ribeye steak: 24 ounces

Porterhouse steak: 24 ounce

Beef (Grounded): 18 ounces

Salmon cutlets: 30 ounces (or other fatty fish)

Trout: 26 ounces

Lamb Chops: 24 ounces

100% pork sausages: 13 ounces

Pork belly: 10 ounces

Pork chops: 12 ounces

Bacon: 12 ounces

Cheese: 1/2 pounds

Butter: 1 pound

Chicken breasts

Week 2 Diet Plan

In week 2 of your carnivore diet, we will eliminate most by products. You can still cook with some butter, though you should not use dairy products such as cheese. Also, during the second week, adjust to rarer meat cuts for your nutritional benefit. You can also introduce organ meats in this week.

Monday

Breakfast: 2 grilled chicken breasts (about 8 ounces)

Lunch: Slow roast topside of beef (12 ounces)

Dinner: 4 fresh lamb chops (12 ounces)

Tuesday

Breakfast: Ground beef patty-grilled (8 ounces)

Lunch: Roast salmon (around 15 ounces)

Dinner: Ribeye steak- grilled (8 ounces) +beef liver (roasted) (around 4 ounces)

Wednesday

Breakfast: 5 slices (about 4 ounces) of bacon and 1-2 (3 ounces) 100% pork sausages

Lunch: Grilled porterhouse steak (12 ounces) with butter

Dinner: Slow roast topside of beef (12 ounces)

Thursday

Breakfast: Ribeye steak-grilled (12 ounces)

Lunch: 3 chicken breasts-grilled with skin (12 ounces)

Dinner: Ground beef burger patty- grilled (12 ounces)

Friday

Breakfast: Grilled steak (about 8 ounces) with some butter

Lunch: Slow roast beef (8 ounces) + roasted beef liver (4 ounces)

Dinner: 4 grilled or fried pork chops (about 12 ounces)

Saturday

Breakfast: Grilled ground beef burger (8 ounces)

Lunch: 15 ounces of roast salmon with butter

Dinner: Grilled sirloin steak (12 ounces)

Sunday

Breakfast: Grilled steak (8 ounces)

Lunch: Slow roast beef (12 ounces)

Dinner: 3 (12 ounces) grilled chicken breasts with skin + 4 ounces of roasted beef liver

Week 3 Diet Plan

During week 3, you need to remove all by-products of milk, and then shift towards eating more beef. You will also eat less of fish and poultry and more of beef. You will also eat more of organ meat.

Monday

Breakfast: 8 ounces of grilled beef burger patty

Lunch: 8 ounces of Slow roast beef + 4 ounces of roast beef liver

Dinner: 15 ounces of Roasted salmon (or any fatty fish) cutlets on the bone

Tuesday

Breakfast: 5 slices (about 4 ounces) of bacon and 1-2 (3 ounces) pork sausages

Lunch: Grilled beef burger patty (12 ounces)

Dinner: Grilled porterhouse steak (about 12 ounces)

Wednesday

Breakfast: Grilled ribeye steak (8 ounces)

Lunch: 12 ounces of Grilled beef burger patty

Dinner: 4 pork chops grilled or fried (12 ounces)

Thursday

Breakfast: Grilled porterhouse steak (8 ounces)

Lunch: 3 grilled chicken breasts with skin (12 ounces)

Dinner: 8 ounces of Slow roast topside of beef + 4 ounces of slow-cooked beef Kidney

Friday

Breakfast: Grilled ground beef burger patty (8 ounces)

Lunch: Grilled ribeye steak (8 ounces) + roasted beef liver (4 ounces)

Dinner: Grilled porterhouse steak (12 ounces)

Saturday

Breakfast: 3 fresh lamb chops (8 ounces)

Lunch: 12 ounces of Grilled ground beef burger patty

Dinner: 12 ounces of Slow roast topside of beef

Sunday

Breakfast: 8 ounces of Grilled ribeye steak

Lunch: 12 ounces of Grilled ground beef burger patty

Dinner: 8 ounces of Slow roast topside of beef + 4 ounces of slow-cooked beef Kidney

Week 4 Diet Plan

During the fourth week, you should only eat beef. You should also include more organ meats. Make sure to purchase only grass-fed beef if your budget allows it; if not, try squeezing in as much grass-fed beef when possible.

Monday

Breakfast: 8 ounces of Grilled Beef burger patty

Lunch: 8 ounces of Slow roast beef + 4 ounces of roast beef liver seasoned with one pinch of salt

Dinner: 24 ounces of BBQ beef ribs (bones included)

Tuesday

Breakfast: Grilled sirloin steak (8 ounces)

Lunch: 12 ounces of BBQ beef burger patty

Dinner: 12 ounces of Grilled porterhouse steak

Wednesday

Breakfast: Grilled ribeye steak (8 ounces)

Lunch: 8 ounces of Grilled beef burger patty + 4 ounces of roast beef liver

Dinner: BBQ sirloin steak (12 ounces)

Thursday

Breakfast: 8 ounces of Grilled porterhouse steak

Lunch: 24 ounces of BBQ beef ribs (bones included)

Dinner: 8 ounces of Slow roast topside of beef + 4 ounces of slow-cooked beef Kidney

Friday

Breakfast: 8 ounces of Grilled ground beef burger patty

Lunch: 12 ounces of BBQ ribeye steak

Dinner: 12 ounces of Grilled porterhouse steak

Saturday

Breakfast: 8 ounces of Grilled ground beef burger patty + 4 ounces of slow-cooked beef Kidney

Lunch: 12 ounces of Slow roast topside of beef

Dinner: 24 ounces of BBQ beef ribs (bones included)

Sunday

Breakfast: Ribeye steak- grilled (8 ounces)

Lunch: 12 ounces of BBQ beef burger patty

Dinner: 8 ounces of Slow roast beef + 4 ounces of slow-cooked beef Kidney

Chapter 9: Carnivore Diet Breakfast Recipes

Meat Lover Omelette

Serves 1

Prep Time: 7 minutes

Total Time: 10 minutes

Ingredients

1-ounce sausage, cooked

1-ounce bacon, cooked

1-ounce deli ham

2 large eggs

1-ounce cheddar cheese- shredded

1 tablespoon of butter

Directions

Crack the eggs into a small bowl, then whisk until well combined.

Add butter to a 10-inch non-stick skillet and melt over medium heat. Once melted, swirl the butter to coat the bottom of the pan. Pour in the egg mix.

When the eggs start cooking, use a spatula to lift the edges gently, then tip the skillet to allow the uncooked part to flow underneath.

Cook until just set for 3 to 4 minutes.

Sprinkle cheese, ham, sausage, and bacon equally onto half of the omelet before folding in half.

Cook until the cheese is melted, for 1 minute.

Serve right away.

Breakfast Casserole

Serves 12

Prep Time: 30 minutes

Cook Time: 35 minutes

Resting Time: 15 minutes

Ingredients

3/4 cup bacon crumbles or 12 slices

1.5 pounds of sausage

12 eggs

2 cups grated cheese

3/4 cup heavy cream

Optional: 2 teaspoons of hot sauce

Directions

Preheat your oven to 350 degrees F. Grease a casserole baking dish (this recipe used 9 x 13 inches).

Crumble the sausage and brown, then drain off.

Warm the crumbles of bacon with the sausage. If you decide to go with fresh bacon, cook, then crumble.

Place the sausage and bacon at the bottom of the prepared casserole. Add a cup of grated cheese over the meats.

Add the heavy cream, 12 eggs, hot sauce, and seasonings, if desired, to a blender, then process until fluffy or simply mix well in a large bowl.

Pour the egg mixture into the casserole dish with the cheese and meats, then top with the remaining cheese.

Bake until a knife comes out clean when inserted in the middle or for 35-40 minutes.

If desired, garnish with onion.

Carnivore Breakfast Muffins

Serves 4

Prep Time: 10 minutes

Cook Time: 20 minutes

Total Time: 30 minutes

Ingredients

8 ounces ground beef

9 large eggs

1 teaspoon salt

Directions

Preheat your oven to 350 degrees F.

Grease a standard size muffin tin.

Add the ground beef to your skillet, then brown over medium-high heat.

In a large bowl, crack the eggs and whisk well. Add salt and the browned meat, then stir until combined.

Portion the mixture equally among the muffin cups filling every cup to ¾ full. Bake until the eggs are set or for 20 minutes.

Remove from the oven, then allow the muffins to cool for 5 minutes.

Loosen the muffins by running a knife over the edges of all cups, then pop them out. Serve right away or place on a wire rack to continue cooling.

Reheat leftovers in the oven or enjoy cold.

Bacon Egg Cups

Serves 12

Prep Time: 5 minutes

Cook Time: 30 minutes

Total Time: 35 minutes

Ingredients

6 slices bacon

12 large eggs

3 ounces shredded cheddar cheese

Directions

Begin by cooking the bacon in the oven or stovetop- in this recipe I baked the oven at 350 degrees in the oven for 30 to 40 minutes. Once ready, let the bacon cool.

Crack one egg into all the 12 muffin cups.

Cut the bacon into ¼ inch pieces, then add one strip to all the egg cups.

Into all egg cups, top with 0.25 oz. of cheddar cheese.

Break the yolks in each cup using a fork, then stir together the contents of the cup gently.

Bake the bacon egg cups at 350 degrees for 25 to 30 minutes.

Egg Muffins

Serves 12

Prep Time: 10 minutes

Cook Time: 25 minutes

Total Time: 35 minutes

Ingredients

1/2 cup diced ham

1/2 cup shredded cheddar cheese

1/2 cup milk

12 eggs

1/4 teaspoon pepper

1/2 teaspoon salt

Directions

Preheat your oven to 375 degrees F. Prepare your muffin tins by spraying with non-stick cooking spray.

Whisk together the milk, eggs, pepper, and salt in a large mixing bowl. Stir in the ham and cheese.

Divide the mixture over 12 prepared muffin tins.

Bake until muffins are set in the center or for about 25 minutes.

Optional Add-Ins

Cooked ground sausage, ground turkey, ground chicken, crumbled bacon or chorizo.

Chapter 10: Carnivore Diet Lunch Recipes

Thick Cut Pan-Seared Pork Chops

Serves 2

Prep Time: 5 minutes

Cook Time: 15 minutes

Total Time: 20 minutes

Ingredients

2 – 4 (1 inch) thick pork chops

4 tablespoons of butter

Salt and pepper

Optional

1 tablespoon of fresh chives minced

2 cloves of garlic minced

Directions

Use paper towels to pat dry your chops.

In a large skillet, melt 2 tablespoons of butter over medium-high heat. Swirl the butter until the bottom of the pan is coated. In the meantime, preheat your broiler.

Create hash marks on your chops, then season with pepper and salt.

Carefully add the meat to the prepared hot skillet, then let it brown for 2-4 minutes.

Once a nice golden crust forms, flip, then add garlic on top. Cook for 2-4 more minutes, then add a generous scoop of the butter left on top of every pork chop. Transfer to the broiler until the meat reaches a temperature of 140 degrees to finish cooking.

Baste the melted butter into the chops after removing from the oven, then cover and let it sit for 2-4 minutes.

Serve hot with a sprinkle of chives.

Carnivore Burgers

Serves 4

Prep time: 1 hour

Cook time: 7 minutes

Ingredients

6 ounces ground beef heart or liver

12 ounces ground lamb

1 pound grass-fed fatty ground beef

4 ounces blue cheese crumbled

1 teaspoon of salt

Directions

Add all the ingredients into a bowl and mix well, then bring to room temperature.

Shape the burgers, then cook on a grill at medium-high heat for about 3 minutes. If you prefer adding your cheese over the top rather than mixing crumbled cheese into your patties, add after flipping the burgers.

If you won't be making chaffles with these, add a touch of butter before topping with cheese or add the butter after removing the burger from the grill if you won't be placing cheese over the top.

Carnivore Braised Short Ribs

Serves 6

Total time: 2 hours 10 minutes

Ingredients

2 cups chicken bone broth

A liberal amount of salt for seasoning

4 pounds of short ribs (about 8 ribs)

Optional: 1 tablespoon garlic sauce

Directions

Preheat your oven to 325° F.

Generously season the ribs on all sides with salt. Let the short ribs stand for a minimum of half an hour so that the meat can absorb the salt.

Into a large Dutch oven, add your preferred cooking fat (duck fat, tallow, lard), then place over medium-high heat until heated. Work in batches where you sear 3 to 4 short ribs for 1-2 minutes per side or until all sides have formed a golden-brown crust.

Working in batches eliminates the steaming effect that can occur if you fill the Dutch oven with meat. Steaming prevents the ribs from developing a nice crust which locks the moisture and flavors inside the meat.

Return the meat into the Dutch oven, then pour in the chicken bone broth and garlic sauce (if desired). Allow the mixture to boil, then turn off the heat.

Place in the oven and bake at 325 degrees F for 1 ½ to 2 hours or until the rib meat is fork-tender and has pulled back from the bone.

Easy Seared Tongue

Serves 3

Prep Time: 25 minutes

Cook Time: 2 hours, 5 minutes

Total Time: 2 hours, 30 minutes

Ingredients

3-4 canoe cut marrow bones, 1 for every serving

Lard, fat of your choice, or bacon grease

Salt

1 beef tongue

Directions

Coat the tongue with salt one day before cooking, then transfer to a container with a lid and fill with water. Place in the fridge overnight.

Rinse the tongue, then transfer to a pot. Pour in water to cover by several inches, then let it boil. If there is any foam rising to the surface, skim it. Adjust the heat to simmer, then secure the lid over the pot. Let the meat simmer for a few hours.

Preserve the skimmed broth to make soup or something else along the week, then transfer the beef tongue to a cutting board or plate. Allow the meat to cool enough to touch before peeling the tongue.

In the meantime, put the marrow bones on your baking sheet, then broil for 10 minutes.

Add lard to a pan, then place over medium heat. Cut the meat into strips, then season with salt if desired. Place in the pan and sear for a few minutes, then flip and sear for another minute to heat through the other side.

Pan-Fried Kidney

Serves 2

Prep Time: 10 minutes

Cook Time: 5 minutes

Total Time: 15 minutes

Ingredients

2 tablespoons of butter

1 cup olive oil

1 pound beef kidney

1 tablespoon each of pepper and salt

1 tablespoon lemon juice

1 cup of flour

Optional

3 garlic cloves, minced

2 teaspoons of ground coriander

Directions

Pull the white lining and trim off the kidney, then slice the organ meat into 1-inch cubes.

Soak the kidney cubes in salted cold water or cold water with a bit of vinegar or lemon juice for 2 hours. Alternatively, they can be blanched for 20 minutes in boiled water with some extra lemon juice or vinegar.

Pat dry using paper towels then season with pepper and salt. Mix well with flour until coated well.

Start to heat the oil in a pan over high heat. Toss in the meat cubes once the butter is hot, then sauté until cooked through. Once ready, remove the meat from the pan.

Add butter, coriander (if using), and garlic to the same pan, then cook until the garlic becomes light brown. Toss the kidney back in, then pour in lemon juice and cook for an extra 30 seconds.

Top with a generous sprinkle of pepper and salt.

Grilled Salmon

Serves 4

Prep Time: 20 minutes

Cook Time: 20 minutes

Resting time: 3 minutes

Total Time: 43 minutes

Ingredients

4 (6-8 ounce) skin-on salmon fillets about 1 inch thick

1 lemon cut into wedges

2 tablespoons grapeseed oil

2 teaspoons freshly ground black pepper

2 teaspoons kosher salt

Directions

Prep your grill to cook directly over high heat, around 450-550 degrees F. Clean the cooking grates by brushing, then secure the lid to heat.

Coat the meaty side of the fillets generously with oil, then evenly season with pepper and salt. Place the salmon on the grill with the skin side facing down, then grill with the lid secured over direct heat. Cook until the fish is firm to the touch, lighter in color, and can be lifted off without sticking, about 6 to 8 minutes.

Flip over the fillets, then secure the lid and cook at 130 degrees F to medium rare for about 2 to 4 minutes. Move the cooked fish to cool in a platter for 1 to 2 minutes. Slide off the skin from the salmon, then serve with lemon wedges and sauce.

Chapter 11: Carnivore Diet Dinner Recipes

Slow Cooker Pork Ribs

Serves 4

Prep Time: 10 minutes

Cook Time: 6 hours

Total Time: 6 hours 10 minutes

Ingredients

1/2 cup apple cider vinegar

1 rack pork ribs

Garlic salt, pepper, and salt, for seasoning

Directions

If desired or necessary, carve off the membrane from the ribs. Do it by sliding your butter knife below the membrane to create a pocket. Slip 2 or 3 fingers below the membrane to make more room. Grip the membrane using a paper towel, then yank it off until it's removed entirely.

Use pepper and salt to season your pork ribs on all sides generously

Add the cider vinegar to your crock pot's liner, followed by the seasoned ribs. Position the pork ribs so that it sits upward, facing the meaty part against the liner to give your meat a crispy golden outside.

Cook for about 6 hours on the low setting.

Pot Roast with Gravy

Serves 4

Prep Time: 10 minutes

Cook Time: 3 hours

Total time: 3 hours 10 minutes

Ingredients

1 (4-5 pounds) pot roast

3-6 cups beef broth

4 tablespoons of butter or ghee divided

2 teaspoons sea salt

Directions

Turn your Instant Pot onto the sauté feature, then melt your butter or ghee.

Toss in the pot roast and allow it to sear for around 2 minutes on each side.

Pour in the broth to fully cover the meat, then secure the lid and ensure the vent is sealed

Cook for 90 minutes on high heat.

Allow the pressure to release naturally, and check that the meat is fork tender.

Transfer the remaining 2 tablespoons of ghee and 1 ½ cups of the broth left to a small saucepan, then heat over medium heat. Constantly stir the contents of the saucepan until the broth is reduced and has thickened, around 5 to 6 minutes.

Serve the pot roast onto a plate, then cut crosswise.

Drizzle the sauce over your roast and enjoy.

Carnivore Casserole with Ground Beef

Serves 4

Prep Time: 5 minutes

Cook Time: 25 minutes

Total Time: 30 minutes

Ingredients

6 large eggs

½ cup heavy cream

1 pound of ground beef

1 teaspoon salt

2 tablespoons cream cheese softened

Directions

Preheat your oven to 350 degrees F.

Cook the ground beef over medium heat in a skillet until lightly browned.

In a large bowl, whisk the eggs. Pour in the cream cheese, salt, and heavy cream, then mix until combined well. Toss in the ground beef and mix well.

Transfer the resulting mixture to a 9 inch round pie plate that is greased. Bake in the oven until the eggs set, around 25-30 minutes.

Allow your casserole to stand for 10 minutes before slicing and serve.

Roast Pork Belly

Serves 8

Prep Time: 10 minutes

Cook Time: 1 hour

Total Time: 1 hour 30 minutes

Ingredients

2 teaspoons olive oil

2 pounds of pork belly

2 teaspoons salt

1/2 teaspoon Pepper

Directions

Preheat your oven to 460 degrees F (240° C).

Carve your pork belly's skin, then use a paper towel to pat it dry.

Use olive oil, pepper, and salt to rub the entire pork belly.

Transfer the meat skin side up to your roasting tray, then bake in the oven until the skin begins blistering, around 25-30 minutes.

Adjust the oven temperature to 320 degrees F (160° C), then continue roasting for 1 hour to 1 hour 15 minutes.

Once ready, remove the pork belly frome the oven, cover using aluminum foil, then let it stand for 20 minutes before you serve.

Organ Meat Pie

Serves 4

Prep Time: 5 minutes

Cook Time: 15 minutes

Total Time: 20 minutes

Ingredients

½ pound ground beef liver

½ pound ground beef heart

½ pound ground beef

3 eggs

Ghee, butter or beef tallow, or other cooking fat melted

Salt

Directions

Preheat your oven to 350 degrees F.

In a mixing bowl, mix all organ meat with salt and then transfer to a skillet and lightly brown over medium-high heat.

In a bowl, whisk the eggs, then drizzle over browned meat. Mix well.

Bake until the eggs set or for 15 to 20 minutes, in a 9 inch cast iron, 8×8-inch baking dish, or a 9-inch pie plate.

Remove from oven, let it cool for five minutes. Enjoy warm and serve any leftovers cold.

Chicken Wrapped in Bacon

Serves 4

Prep Time: 5 minutes

Cook Time: 45 minutes

Total Time: 50 minutes

Ingredients

300 g Bacon

1 kg Chicken Thigh (With Bone and Skin)

1 teaspoon of Salt

Directions

Preheat your oven to 200 degrees F. Coat your bacon in salt, then put the chicken thighs skin side down over the strips.

Turn over the chicken, then fold the tips of your bacon beneath.

Bake until the bacon appears all nice and crispy or for about 45 to 60 minutes.

Chapter 12: Carnivore Diet Appetizers, Snacks, and Sides

Pizza Pie

Serves 4

Prep Time: 2 minutes

Cooking Time: 15 minutes

Total Time: 17 minutes

Ingredients

3 large organic eggs

1 pound double-ground veal

10 thin slices of smoked beef prosciutto

3.5 ounces crumbled Greek Feta

½ teaspoon of butter or tallow for the pan

1.8 ounces grated aged goat or sheep's cheese

Directions

Use your hands to mix the minced meat with crumbled feta cheese and eggs.

Prepare the clay or ceramic pie pan by greasing it with butter or tallow.

Transfer the mixture to the prepared pan, then tap to form a pizza-like crust and cover the pan.

Layer the smoked beef slices over the top, then sprinkle with the cheese.

Bake for 15 minutes in your oven at 400°F. If your oven features an upper roasting setting, roast the carnivore pie for 1 minute with the higher heater set to maximum to develop a crispy golden result.

Recipe Notes

You can make this meat pie using ground goat or lamb. If you use beef, it takes a longer time to cook and may not turn out to be soft when it cools.

Chicken Tenderloins with Bacon

Serves 5

Prep Time:5 minutes

Cook Time:20 minutes

Total Time: 25 minutes

Ingredients

Bacon-Wrapped Chicken Nuggets

10 slices bacon

10 pieces chicken tenderloins or strips

Optional Sauce

Double/heavy cream, enough to make the sauce and deglaze pan

50 g (1.8 ounces) cream cheese full fat

Directions

Use a streaky slice of bacon to wrap all chicken tenderloins.

There are 2 ways to cook these. Either transfer to a baking dish, then bake for 20 minutes at 350F, or transfer to a frying pan and fry gently until golden on all sides for about 15 minutes.

Take out the wrapped meats from the pan/baking dish, then deglaze to pick the flavor of bacon. Create a creamy sauce by adding the cream cheese. Ensure that the cream you add is sufficient to create a pourable sauce.

Brown Butter Steak Bites

Serves 3

Prep Time: 3 minutes

Cook Time: 14 minutes

Total Time: 17 minutes

Ingredients

3 tablespoons good quality salted butter

1 pound sirloin steak, cut into cubes

2-3 tablespoons water

1-2 teaspoons kosher salt

1 tablespoon olive oil

Directions

Place a large cast-iron or stainless steel skillet/pan over high heat. It's possible to use non-stick though it won't give you the same sear on your steak. Sprinkle the cubes of steak with salt, then toss until all sides are coated.

Add in the oil once the skillet heats through for a couple of minutes. The oil should shimmer over the surface if the pan is scorching enough.

Add the sirloin bites into the skillet in one layer without overlapping. Cook until a crusty sear forms, for about 3 to 4 minutes, without flipping or stirring. Once the crust has formed, turn over all the bites one at a time to brown the other side well.

Transfer the steak bites from the skillet, then place aside to stand. Adjust the heat to medium-low, then deglaze the pan by adding water. This loosens all the crispy bits that have formed on the pan's surface and ensures that they are included in the sauce.

Add butter to the skillet once the water evaporates. Slightly toast the butter until milk solids begin browning, about 5 to 7 minutes. You should notice golden brown flecks developing and smell a nutty fragrance. Reduce the heat if your butter starts smoking.

Toss back the pieces of steak into the skillet for 1-2 minutes to coat in butter, then serve right away.

Carnivore Chicken Nuggets

Yields 60 Nuggets

Prep Time: 40 minutes

Cook Time: 20 minutes

Total Time: 1 hour

Ingredients

Chicken Mixture

3 pounds ground chicken

1/2 teaspoon of pink salt

1 large egg

Optional: 1 /2 teaspoon oregano

Breading Mixture

1 cup parmesan cheese grated

1 cup pork rinds ground

Directions

Preheat your oven to 400° F and prepare your cookie sheet by lining using parchment paper.

In a flat container, mix the cheese and pork rinds.

Mix the egg, spices, and chicken in another container.

Use the resulting chicken mix to create a small-sized patty of your preferred size. Put the patty on the breading mixture, then coat using a fork.

Transfer to the prepared cookie sheet, then repeat the previous step until you have used all the chicken mixture. If the breading runs out, just make more.

Bake for 20 minutes at 400° F.

Carnivore Pizza Crust

Serves 4

Prep Time: 5 minutes

Cook Time: 25 minutes

Additional Time: 5 minutes

Total Time: 35 minutes

Ingredients

Carnivore Pizza Crust

1 pound extra-lean ground chicken

1 cup ground pork rinds

1 tablespoon Italian seasoning

¼ teaspoon each of pepper and salt

Pizza Toppings

For Carnivore: Cheese and Pepperoni are perfect!

Directions

Preheat your oven to 425 degrees F.

Prepare 2 large rimmed baking sheets by lining with parchment paper.

Add all ingredients to a large bowl, then mix with a fork until well-combined.

Transfer the resulting mixture to a wax paper sheet and cover using another sheet. Mold using your hands to the desired shape (if you like, you could separate the mixture to make two pizzas).

Flatten the mixture as much as possible using a rolling pin, then peel off the wax paper. Transfer the crust to the prepared baking sheet carefully; use a spatula to trim and repair edges.

Bake until edges start to turn brown and curl for about 25 minutes at 425 degrees F.

Once cooking time is up, take the crust out of the oven, then set the oven to broil.

Add your desired carnivore-friendly toppings over the crust, then broil until the toppings brown and the cheese is melted, about 5 minutes.

Enjoy!

Homemade Beef Jerky

Serves 6

Prep Time:10 minutes

Cook Time:1 hour 30 minutes

Total Time:1 hour 40 minutes

Ingredients

4 tablespoons of butter, lard, or duck fat

300g beef

Salt and cracked pepper to taste

Optional: natural spices to taste

Directions

Prepare your baking sheet by lining it with parchment or non-stick baking paper.

Cut the meat into slim strips, 1 to 2cm in width.

Transfer the beef strips to a bowl with your preferred spices and enough melted butter to cover the meat. Toss the beef to coat with spices and butter.

Layer the beef strips onto the prepared baking sheet, then bake for an hour at 80 degrees C. Flip over all jerky strips, then continue baking for an extra 30 minutes.

Switch off your oven, then leave the beef jerky to rest in the dry, warm oven.

Store in an airtight container for up to two weeks.

Carnivore Beef Liver Pâté

Serves 2

Prep Time: 45 minutes

Cook Time: 8 minutes

Total Time: 53 minutes

Ingredients

2 tablespoons of heavy cream

50 g grass-fed butter

250 g beef liver or lamb

Optional: 1/2 teaspoon of thyme

Directions

Transfer the liver to a bowl, then cover it with brine or salted water. Place in the refrigerator for 45 minutes.

Remove liver from saltwater and pat dry using paper towels. Place your frying pan over medium heat, then melt the butter. Toss in the liver and brown for 5 minutes on either side.

Add the butter and liver (along with thyme if using) to a blender or food processor, then process to achieve a smooth texture. Add in heavy cream and blend once more.

Spoon the resulting mixture into 2 ramekins and cover the tops with foil. Place in the refrigerator for 2 hours before serving.

Liver Meatballs

Serves 8

Prep Time: 20 minutes

Cook Time: 5 minutes

Ingredients

2 egg yolks pasture-raised

2 pounds ground beef grass-fed

10 ounces bacon uncured

1 pound beef liver grass-fed

Pepper and salt to taste

Optional: 1 yellow onion

Other desired natural spices to taste

Directions

Cook your bacon over medium heat until done. Try making your bacon crispier as it slightly affects the texture and taste of the final meal. Keep the lard from bacon.

Transfer the cooked bacon to your food processor, then pulse until the bacon has crumbled.

Cut your liver into chunks, then pour into the food processor. Blend until the bacon and liver are processed into a coarse paste. When you over blend, the liver liquefies, and you won't like that.

In a mixing bowl, mix the bacon liver mixture with the egg yolk, spices, and ground beef using a spoon. If desired, dice the onion and add it here.

If your mixture turns out to be too wet to form patties or meatballs easily, place it in the fridge for a while to make it easy to handle and form balls.

Parmesan-Pork Meatballs

Serves 4

Prep Time: 5 minutes

Cook Time: 45 minutes

Total Time: 50 minutes

Ingredients

2 pounds ground pork

2 eggs (optional)

1 cup of shredded parmesan cheese

1 teaspoon sea salt

Directions

Add the eggs (if desired), cheese, and ground pork to a bowl and mix until combined well. Adjust the salt a teaspoon at a time.

Preheat your broiler to high. Position the rack to the middle slot from the top. Line with parchment paper a metal baking tray that has shallow sides.

Form meatballs into your preferred size, then transfer to the prepared baking sheet, making sure they make contact but aren't overlapping in any way. For the meatballs to cook evenly, ensure you make them all in the same size.

Place the meatballs in the broiler once preheated and broil until the tops begin darkening, about 5 minutes. If you'd like to freeze your meatballs, take them out now, then cool before transferring them to a freezer-safe bag. Finish cooking from thawed by broiling at 350 degrees F until cooked through, for 20 minutes.

Transfer the meatballs to the center of your oven and set to cook at 350 degrees for 15 to 20 more minutes- depending on the size of your meatballs.

Slice the meatball in half to check for doneness. If slight pink, that's good since the cooking process continues as they cool.

Serve right away and top with more cream sauce or cheese if desired.

Conclusion

The carnivore diet is an amazing diet that ensures you enjoy flavorful meat while enjoying the benefits that this diet has to offer. With all the information I have provided on how the diet works, which foods to eat and avoid, how to get started, carnivore diet meal plan, and the various recipes, you should have an easy and fun time adopting to this way of life.

Good luck and All the best in your journey!

Made in United States
Orlando, FL
12 July 2025

62912695R00046